The Greatest Dash Diet Slow Cooker Cooking Plan

Breakfast, Sides, Soups and Stews.
All in This Complete Cookbook

Carmela Rojas

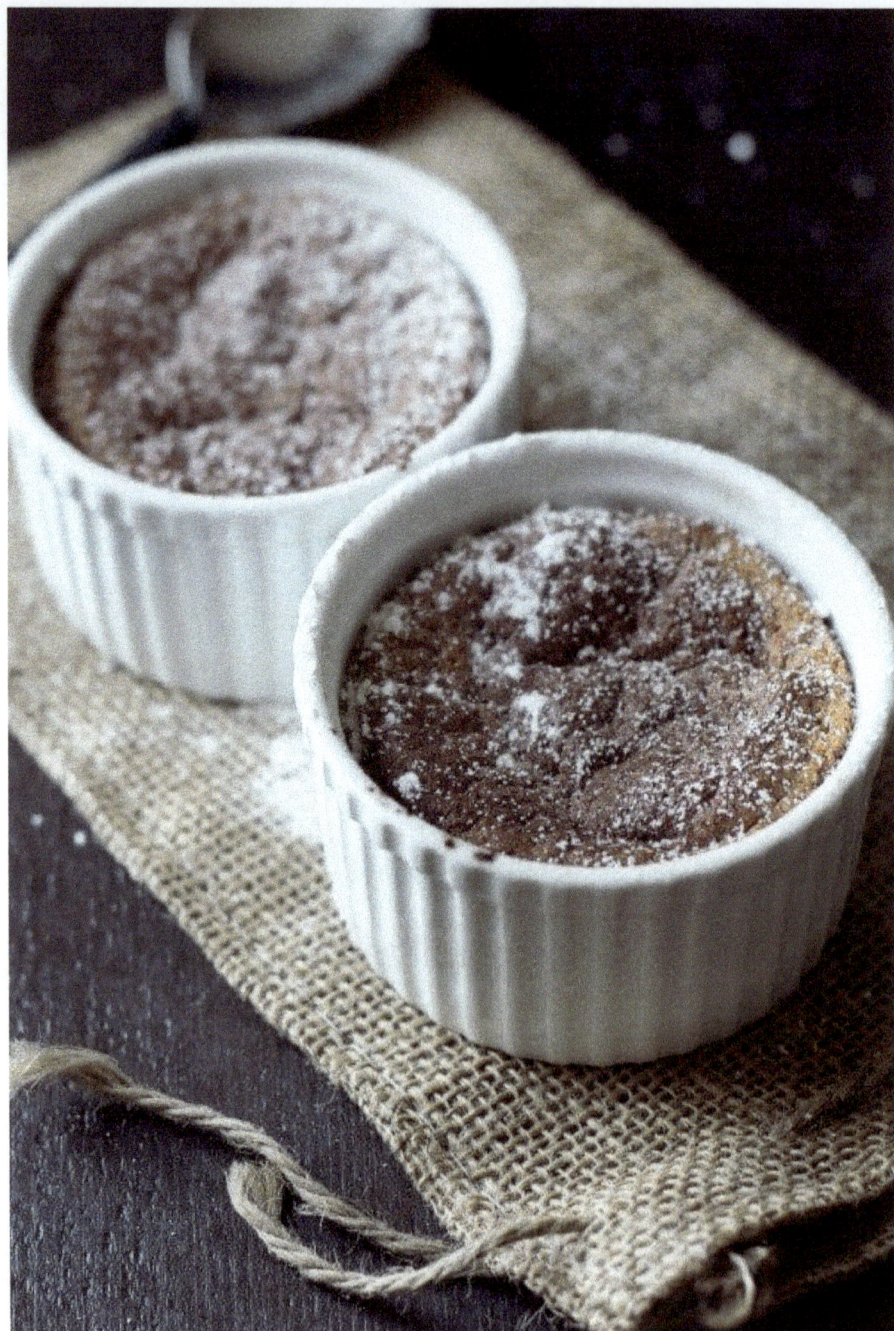

TABLE OF CONTENTS

Spiced Pumpkin Butter

Servings: 8

Cooking Time: 4 Hours

Ingredients:

- 2 teaspoon lemon juice
- 30 ounces pumpkin puree
- ½ cup apple cider
- 1 teaspoon ginger, grated
- 1 teaspoon cinnamon powder
- 1 cup coconut sugar
- 1 teaspoon vanilla extract
- ¼ teaspoon cloves, ground
- ¼ teaspoon allspice, ground
- 1 teaspoon nutmeg, ground

Directions:

1. In your slow cooker, mix pumpkin puree with apple cider, coconut sugar, vanilla extract, cinnamon, nutmeg, lemon juice, ginger, cloves and allspice, stir, cover and cook on Low for 4 hours.
2. Blend using an immersion blender and serve for breakfast.

Nutrition Info:

Calories 60, Fat 0.5g, Cholesterol 0mg, Sodium 11mg, Carbohydrate 13.3g, Fiber 3.2g, Sugars 5.4g, Protein 1.4g, Potassium 245mg

Rolled Oats With Dates

Servings: 4

Cooking Time: 7 Hours

Ingredients:

- 1 cup dates, dried and chopped
- 1 cup walnuts, chopped
- 4 cups water
- 3 cups rolled oats
- 1 teaspoon cloves, ground
- 1 tablespoon ginger, ground
- 1 teaspoon turmeric powder
- 3 cups whole grain cereal flakes
- 1 cup apples, dried and chopped
- 2 tablespoons cinnamon powder
- 1 cup coconut sugar

Directions:

1. In your slow cooker, mix the water with the oats, cereal flakes, apples, dates, walnuts, cinnamon, sugar, cloves, ginger and turmeric, cover and cook on Low for 7 hours.
2. Divide into bowls and serve.

Nutrition Info:

Calories 946, Fat 24.6g, Cholesterol 0mg, Sodium 658mg, Carbohydrate 168.8g, Fiber 23.7g, Sugars 57.7g, Protein 23.9g, Potassium 1077mg

Scallions Quinoa

Servings: 4

Cooking Time: 2 Hours

Ingredients:

- 2 cups low-sodium veggie stock
- ½ cup scallions, chopped
- 1 cup cherry tomatoes, halved
- 1 and ½ cups quinoa
- A pinch of black pepper

Directions:

1. In your slow cooker, combine the quinoa with the tomatoes and the other ingredients, put the lid on and cook on Low for 2 hours.
2. Divide into bowls and serve for breakfast.

Nutrition Info:

Calories 254, Fat .4g, Cholesterol 0mg, Sodium 78mg, Carbohydrate 44.6g, Fiber 5.3g, Sugars 2g, Protein 9.6g, Potassium 500mg

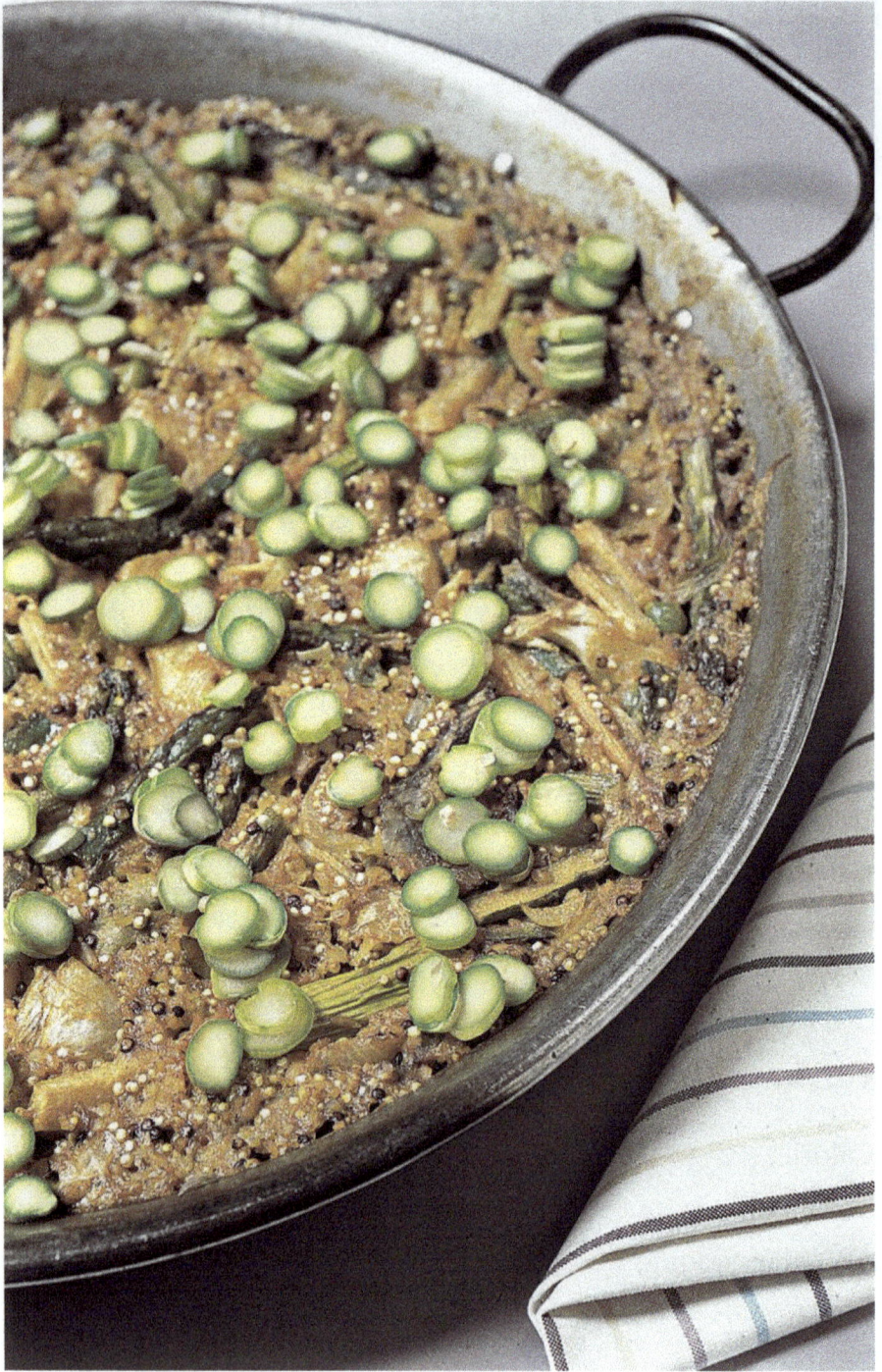

Vanilla Oats With Raisins

Servings: 4

Cooking Time: 6 Hours

Ingredients:

- 2 cups almond milk
- ½ teaspoon cinnamon powder
- 1 tablespoon low-fat butter
- 2 tablespoons stevia
- 2 drops vanilla extract
- Cooking spray
- 1 cup apple, chopped
- ¼ cup raisins
- 1 cup old-fashioned oats

Directions:

1. Grease your slow cooker with the cooking spray, add milk, stevia, butter, cinnamon and vanilla and stir.
2. Add oats, apples and raisins, cover and cook on Low for 7 hours.
3. Divide into bowls and serve.

Nutrition Info:

Calories 437, Fat 43.9g, Cholesterol 350mg, Sodium 1072mg, Carbohydrate 12.5g, Fiber 0.8g, Sugars 3.8g, Protein 34.6g, Potassium 477mg

Rum Raisin Bananas

Servings: 4 Servings

Ingredients:

- 3 tablespoons (45 ml) dark rum, divided
- ¼ cup (35 g) raisins
- 3 tablespoons (42 g) unsalted butter
- ¼ cup (60 g) brown sugar
- 4 bananas
- ¼ teaspoon nutmeg
- ¼ teaspoon cinnamon

Directions:

1. Pour 2 tablespoons (30 ml) of the rum over the raisins in a bowl and set aside. Place the butter, brown sugar, and remaining 1 tablespoon (15 ml) rum in the slow cooker. Turn to high and cook until butter and sugar have melted. Peel the bananas and cut in half lengthwise. Place in the cooker. Cover and cook for 30 minutes, turning halfway through the time. Pour the reserved rum and raisins over the bananas and cook 10 minutes longer. Combine nutmeg and cinnamon and sprinkle over bananas before serving.

Nutrition Info:

Per serving: 95 g water; 284 calories (29% from fat, 2% from protein, 68% from carb); 2 g protein; 9 g total fat; 6 g saturated fat; 2 g monounsaturated fat; 0 g polyunsaturated fat; 47 g carb; 3 g fiber; 33 g sugar; 42 mg phosphorus; 27 mg calcium; 1 mg iron; 9 mg sodium; 532 mg potassium; 338 IU vitamin A; 71 mg ATE vitamin E; 10 mg vitamin C; 23 mg cholesterol

Vanilla Poached Strawberries

Servings: 10

Cooking Time: 3 Hours

Ingredients:

- 4 cups coconut sugar
- 2 tablespoons lemon juice
- 2 pounds strawberries
- 1 cup water
- 1 teaspoon vanilla extract
- 1 teaspoon cinnamon powder

Directions:

1. In your slow cooker, mix strawberries with water, coconut sugar, lemon juice, cinnamon and vanilla, stir, cover, cook on Low for 3 hours, divide into bowls and serve cold.

Nutrition Info:

Calories 69, Fat 0.3g, Cholesterol 0mg, Sodium 18mg, Carbohydrate 14.7g, Fiber 1.8g, Sugars 4.6g, Protein 1g, Potassium 143mg

Red Onion Casserole

Servings: 6

Cooking Time: 4 Hours

Ingredients:

- Black pepper to the taste
- 12 eggs, whisked
- 1 cup baby bell mushrooms, sliced
- 2 cups spinach
- ½ cup low-fat milk
- 1 tablespoon red onion, chopped
- 1 teaspoon garlic, minced

Directions:

1. In a bowl, mix the eggs with black pepper, milk, onion, garlic, mushrooms and spinach, toss, pour into your slow cooker, cover and cook on Low for 4 hours.
2. Slice, divide between plates and serve.

Nutrition Info:

Calories 162, Fat .10g, Cholesterol 328mg, Sodium 328mg, Carbohydrate 5.6g, Fiber 0.5g, Sugars 3.6g, Protein 12.6g, Potassium 246mg

Bread Pudding

Servings: 4 Servings

Ingredients:

- ½ cup (120 ml) egg substitute
- 2¼ cups (535 ml) milk
- 1 teaspoon vanilla
- ½ teaspoon cinnamon
- 2 cups (100 g) bread cubes
- ½ cup (115 g) brown sugar
- ½ cup (75 g) raisins

Directions:

1. Combine all ingredients and pour into 1½-quart (4 L) baking dish. Place metal trivet or crumpled foil in bottom of slow cooker. Add ½ cup (120 ml) hot water to cooker. Set baking dish on trivet or foil. Cover and cook on high for about 2 hours.

Nutrition Info:

Per serving: 156 g water; 303 calories (7% from fat, 14% from protein, 79% from carb); 11 g protein; 2 g total fat; 1 g saturated fat; 1 g monounsaturated fat; 1 g polyunsaturated fat; 62 g carb; 2

g fiber; 46 g sugar; 222 mg phosphorus; 238 mg calcium; 2 mg iron; 137 mg sodium; 590 mg potassium; 395 IU vitamin A; 84 mg ATE vitamin E; 1 mg vitamin C; 3 mg cholesterol

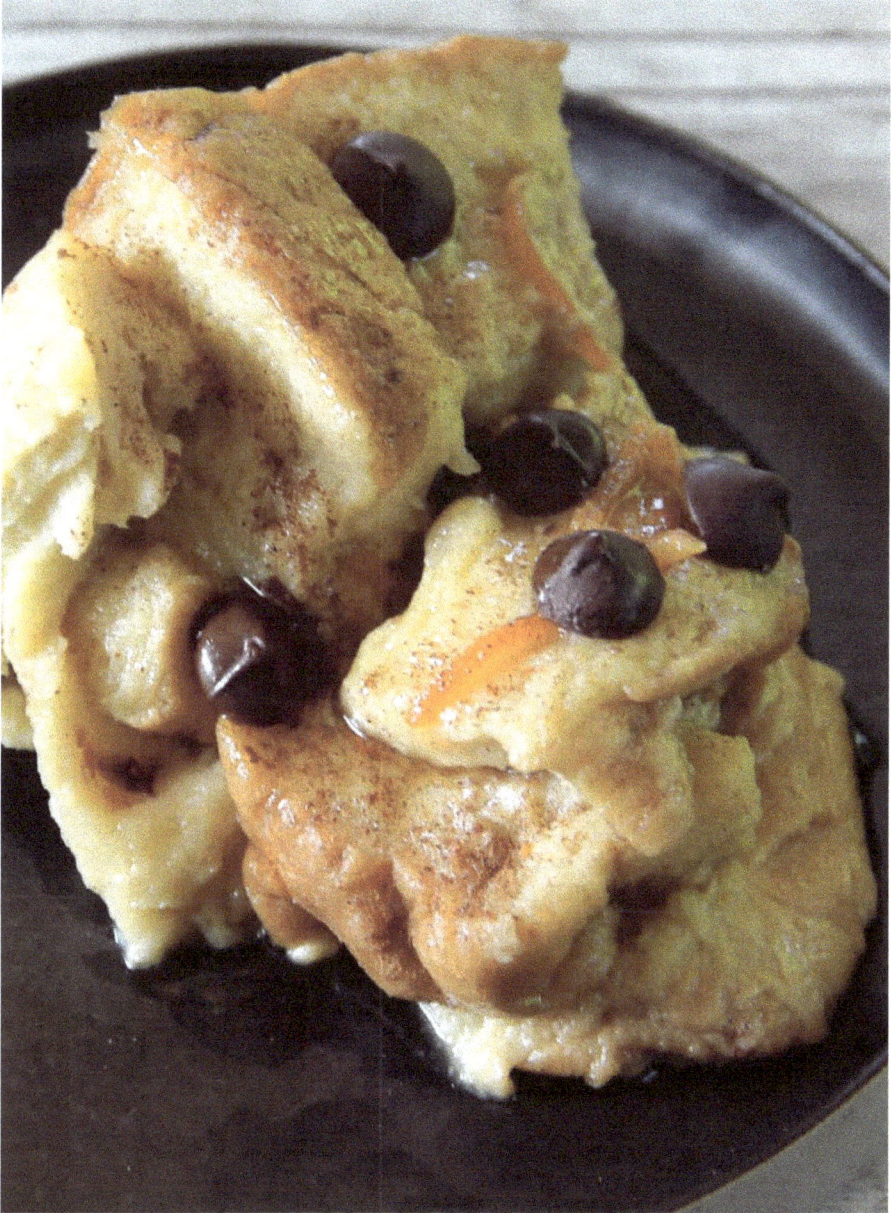

Peaches Compote

Servings: 4

Cooking Time: 4 Hours

Ingredients:
- 2 tablespoons white wine vinegar
- 2 tablespoons lemon juice
- 2 cups blueberries
- ½ cup palm sugar
- 2 peaches, pitted, peeled and cut into wedges
- ½ teaspoon lemon zest, grated
- 1 and ½ cups blackberries
- 1 and ½ cups raspberries

Directions:
1. In your slow cooker, mix blueberries with sugar, vinegar, lemon juice and lemon zest, cover and cook on Low for 4 hours.
2. Divide this into 4 bowl, top with raspberries, blackberries and peach wedges and serve for breakfast.

Nutrition Info:

Calories 273, Fat 0.9g, Cholesterol 0mg, Sodium 1831mg, Carbohydrate 61.9g, Fiber 6g, Sugars 54.2g, Protein 1.8g, Potassium 1857mg

Baked Apples

Servings: 6 Servings

Ingredients:

- 2 tablespoons (18 g) raisins
- ½ cup (100 g) sugar
- 6 apples, cored but left whole and unpeeled
- 1 teaspoon cinnamon
- 2 tablespoons (28 g) unsalted butter
- ¼ cup (60 ml) water

Directions:

1. Mix raisins and sugar together in a small bowl. Stand apples on bottom of slow cooker. Spoon raisin-sugar mixture into centers of apples, dividing evenly among apples. Sprinkle stuffed apples with cinnamon. Dot with butter. Pour the water along the edge of the cooker. Cover and cook on low 3 to 5 hours or on high 2½ to 3½ hours until apples are tender but not collapsing.

Nutrition Info:

Per serving: 122 g water; 237 calories (15% from fat, 1% from protein, 85% from carb); 1 g protein; 4 g total fat; 2 g saturated fat; 1 g monounsaturated fat; 0 g polyunsaturated fat; 53 g carb; 2 g fiber; 49 g sugar; 19 mg phosphorus; 15 mg calcium; 0 mg iron; 1 mg sodium; 145 mg potassium; 168 IU vitamin A; 32 mg ATE vitamin E; 5 mg vitamin C; 10 mg cholesterol

Tasty Cauliflower

Servings: 4

Cooking Time: 6 Hrs 15 Mins

Ingredients:

- 2 minced cloves Garlic
- 2 cups Cauliflower florets
- 2 tbsp. Olive Oil
- Pinch of Sea Salt
- ¼ tsp. Pepper Flakes (chili)
- Pinch of Black Pepper (cracked)
- 4 tbsp. Water
- Zest of ½ lemon

Directions:

1. In a slow cooker, place cauliflower and oil.
2. Add vinegar.
3. Toss well to coat thoroughly.
4. Put in the rest of the ingredients and toss again.
5. Cook on "low" for 2 hrs. Serve immediately.

Nutrition Info:

(Estimated Amount Per Serving): 150 Calories; 14 g Total Fats; 69 mg Sodium; 6 g Carbohydrates; 3 g Dietary Fiber; 2.2 g Protein

Cranberries And Mushroom Bowl

Servings: 12

Cooking Time: 2 Hours And 30 Minutes

Ingredients:

- 1 pound mushrooms, sliced
- 1 cup cranberries, dried
- 6 celery ribs, chopped
- 1 cup cauliflower florets, chopped
- 1 cup low-sodium veggie stock
- 2 yellow onions, chopped
- 2 garlic cloves, minced
- 1 tablespoon sage, chopped
- 1 tablespoons olive oil

Directions:

1. Add the oil to your slow cooker, add mushrooms, celery, onion, garlic, sage, cranberries, cauliflower and stock, stir, cover and cook on High for 2 hours and 30 minutes.
2. Divide between plates and serve as a side dish.

Nutrition Info:

Calories 46, Fat 1.6g, Cholesterol 0mg, Sodium 40mg, Carbohydrate 6.3g, Fiber 2g, Sugars 2.8g, Protein 2.1g, Potassium 292mg

Pepper And Corn Salad

Servings: 6

Cooking Time: 2 Hours

Ingredients:

- 2 ounces prosciutto, cut into strips
- 1 teaspoon olive oil
- 2 cups corn
- ½ cup salt-free tomato sauce
- 1 green bell pepper, chopped
- 1 teaspoon garlic, minced

Directions:

1. Grease your slow cooker with the oil, add corn, prosciutto, tomato sauce, garlic and bell pepper, cover and cook on High for 2 hours.
2. Divide between plates and serve as a side dish.

Nutrition Info:

Calories 79, Fat 1.9g, Cholesterol 5mg, Sodium 130mg, Carbohydrate 13.5g, Fiber 2.1g, Sugars 3.9g, Protein 4.2g, Potassium 274mg

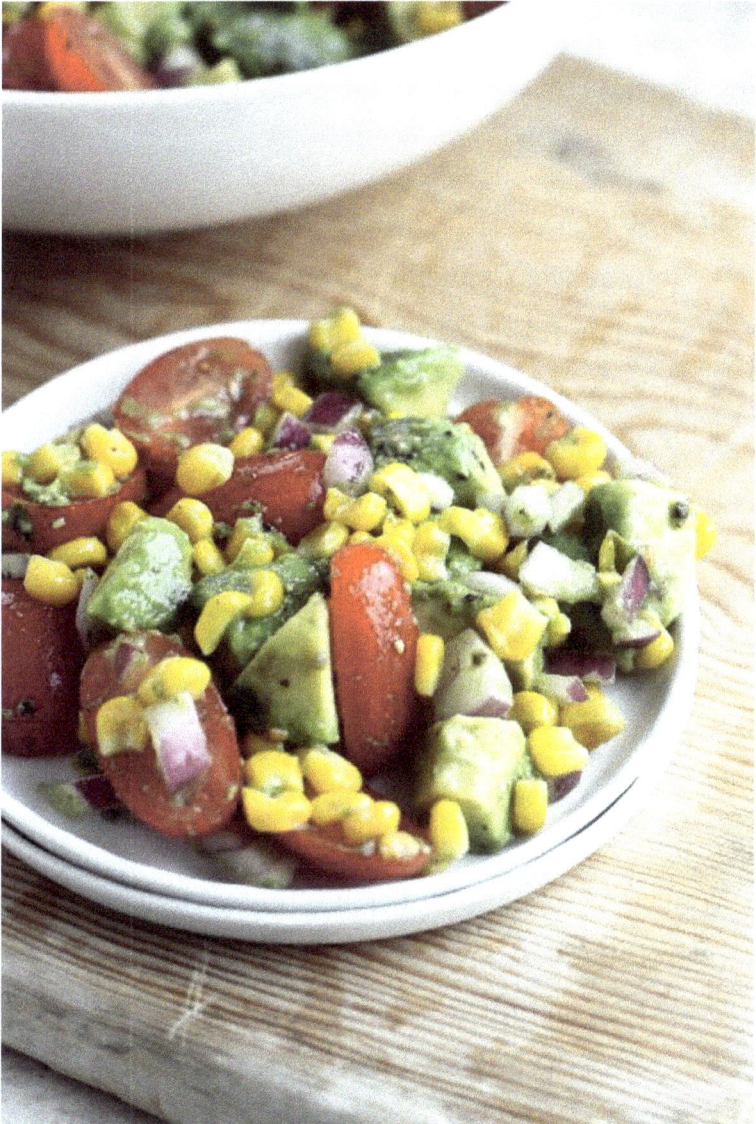

Bean Spread

Servings: About 20

Cooking Time: 4 Hrs

Ingredients:

- 30 ounces Cannellini Beans
- ½ cup Broth (chicken or veg)
- 1 tbsp. Olive Oil
- 3 minced cloves Garlic
- ½ tsp. Marjoram
- ½ tsp. Rosemary
- 1/8 tsp. Pepper
- Pita Chips
- 1 tblsp. Olive Oil

Directions:

1. Place olive oil, beans, broth, marjoram, garlic, rosemary and pepper in the slow cooker.
2. Cook on "low" for 4 hrs.
3. Mash the mixture and transfer to a bowl.
4. Serve with Pita.

Nutrition Info:

(Estimated Amount Per Serving): 298 Calories; 18 g Total Fat; 10 mg Cholesterol; 298 mg Sodium; 30 mg Carbohydrates; 3 g Dietary Fiber; 19 g Protein

Garam Masala Cauliflower

Servings: 4

Cooking Time: 4 Hours

Ingredients:

- 1 pound cauliflower florets
- 2 teaspoons avocado oil
- 1 cup coconut cream
- ½ teaspoon garam masala
- 3 garlic cloves, minced
- ½ teaspoon ginger, ground
- Black pepper to the taste
- ¼ cup chives, chopped

Directions:

1. In your slow cooker, combine the cauliflower with the oil, cream and the other ingredients, put the lid on and cook on Low for 4 hours.
2. Divide between plates and serve as a side dish.

Nutrition Info:

Calories 207, Fat 16.3g, Cholesterol 0mg, Sodium 324mg, Carbohydrate 14.7g, Fiber 4.6g, Sugars 7.1g, Protein 4.2g, Potassium 530mg

Parsley Red Potatoes

Servings: 8

Cooking Time: 6 Hours

Ingredients:
- 16 baby red potatoes, halved
- 2 cups low-sodium chicken stock
- 1 carrot, sliced
- 1 celery rib, chopped
- ¼ cup yellow onion, chopped
- 1 tablespoon parsley, chopped
- 2 tablespoons olive oil
- A pinch of black pepper
- 1 garlic clove minced

Directions:
1. In your slow cooker, mix the potatoes with the carrot, celery, onion, stock, parsley, garlic, oil and black pepper, toss, cover and cook on Low for 6 hours.
2. Divide between plates and serve as a side dish.

Nutrition Info:

Calories 257, Fat 9.5g, Cholesterol 0mg, Sodium 845mg, Carbohydrate 43.4g, Fiber 4.4g, Sugars 4.6g, Protein 4.4g, Potassium 47mg

Cumin Brussels Sprouts

Servings: 4

Cooking Time: 3 Hours

Ingredients:

- 1 cup low-sodium veggie stock
- 1 pound Brussels sprouts, trimmed and halved
- 1 teaspoon rosemary, dried
- 1 teaspoon cumin, ground
- 1 tablespoon mint, chopped

Directions:

1. In your slow cooker, combine the sprouts with the stock and the other ingredients, put the lid on and cook on Low for 3 hours.
2. Divide between plates and serve as a side dish.

Nutrition Info:

Calories 56, Fat 0.6g, Cholesterol 0mg, Sodium 65mg, Carbohydrate 11.4g, Fiber 4.5g, Sugars 2.7g, Protein 4g, Potassium 460mg

Chili Powder Sprouts Salad

Servings: 4

Cooking Time: 2 Hours

Ingredients:

- 1 pound baby spinach
- ½ pound Brussels sprouts, trimmed and halved
- 2 teaspoons avocado oil
- 1 red onion, sliced
- ½ teaspoon chili powder
- 2 tomatoes, cubed
- ½ cup low sodium veggie stock
- Black pepper to the taste

Directions:

1. In your slow cooker, combine the spinach with the sprouts, oil and the other ingredients, put the lid on and cook on High for 2 hours.
2. Divide the mix between plates and serve as a side dish.

Nutrition Info:

Calories 111, Fat 2.6g, Cholesterol 0mg, Sodium 440mg, Carbohydrate 19.3g, Fiber 6.3g, Sugars 6.9g, Protein 6.3g, Potassium 1053mg

Zucchini With Fennel Seeds

Servings: 4

Cooking Time: 3 Hours

Ingredients:

- 1 pound eggplants, roughly cubed
- 1 teaspoon fennel seeds, crushed
- ½ teaspoon rosemary, dried
- 2 tablespoons red curry paste
- ½ teaspoon curry powder
- 1 tablespoon olive oil
- 1 garlic clove, minced
- A pinch of black pepper
- 1 and ½ cups coconut cream
- 1 tablespoon parsley, chopped

Directions:

1. In the slow cooker, combine the eggplants with the crushed fennel rosemary and the other ingredients, put the lid on and cook on Low for 3 hours.
2. Divide the eggplant mix between plates and serve.

Nutrition Info:

Calories 300, Fat 27.5g, Cholesterol 0mg, Sodium 407mg, Carbohydrate 14g, Fiber 6.4g, Sugars 6.4g, Protein 3.4g, Potassium 519mg

Sweet And Sour Red Cabbage

Servings: 6 Servings

Ingredients:

- 4 cups (280 g) shredded red cabbage
- 1 cup (160 g) chopped onion
- 1 cup (150 g) peeled and chopped apple
- ½ cup (115 g) brown sugar
- ½ cup (120 ml) cider vinegar

Directions:

1. Place vegetables in a slow cooker. Combine sugar and vinegar, pour over vegetables, and stir to mix. Cook on low for 7 to 8 hours.

Nutrition Info:

Per serving: 112 g water; 111 calories (1% from fat, 4% from protein, 95% from carb); 1 g protein; 0 g total fat; 0 g saturated fat; 0 g monounsaturated fat; 0 g polyunsaturated fat; 27 g carb; 2 g fiber; 23 g sugar; 33 mg phosphorus; 51 mg calcium; 1 mg iron; 25 mg sodium; 278 mg potassium; 670 IU vitamin A; 0 mg ATE vitamin E; 37 mg vitamin C; 0 mg cholesterol

Spinach And Chickpeas Mix

Servings: 6

Cooking Time: 8 Hours

Ingredients:

- 30 ounces canned chickpeas, no-salt-added, drained and rinsed
- 28 ounces low-sodium veggie stock
- 4 cups baby spinach
- 8 ounces zucchini, sliced
- A pinch of black pepper
- 2 cups cherry tomatoes, halved
- 2 garlic cloves, minced
- 1 cup corn
- 7 small baby carrots
- 2 tablespoons olive oil
- 2 tablespoons rosemary, chopped

Directions:

1. In your slow cooker, mix chickpeas with oil, rosemary, pepper, cherry tomatoes, garlic, corn, baby carrots, zucchini, spinach and stock, stir, cover, cook on Low for 8 hours, divide between plates and serve.

44

Nutrition Info:

Calories 617, Fat 14g, Cholesterol 0mg, Sodium 147mg, Carbohydrate 98.2g, Fiber 27.8g, Sugars 19.4g, Protein 29.9g, Potassium 1705mg

Creamy Zucchini Casserole

Servings: 6 Servings

Ingredients:

- 3 cups (360 g) thinly sliced zucchini
- 1 cup (160 g) diced onion
- 1 cup (130 g) shredded carrot
- 10 ounces (280 g) low-sodium cream of mushroom soup
- 10 ounces (280 g) low-sodium cream of chicken soup

Directions:

1. Spray slow cooker with nonstick cooking spray. Mix vegetables and soups together gently in slow cooker. Cover and cook on high 4 to 6 hours or until vegetables are as crunchy or as soft as you like.

Nutrition Info:

Per serving: 184 g water; 78 cal (19% from fat, 12% from protein, 69% from carb); 2 g protein; 2 g total fat; 1 g saturated fat; 0 g monounsaturated fat; 1 g polyunsaturated fat; 14 g carb; 2 g fiber; 5 g sugar; 87 mg phosphorus; 35 mg calcium; 1 mg iron; 52 mg sodium; 623 mg potassium; 3718 IU vitamin A; 2 mg ATE vitamin E; 14 mg vitamin C; 3 mg Cholesterol

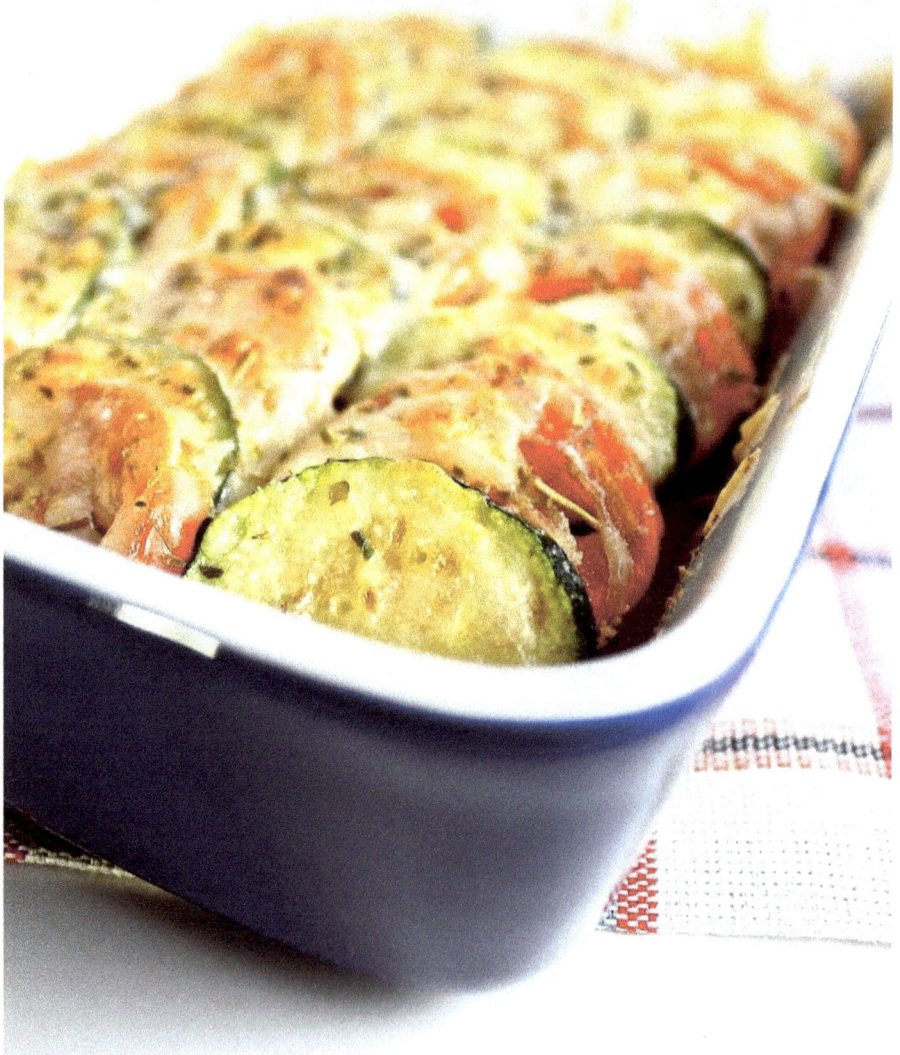

Peach And Carrots

Servings: 6

Cooking Time: 6 Hours

Ingredients:

- 2 pounds small carrots, peeled
- ½ cup low-fat butter, melted
- ½ cup canned peach, unsweetened
- 2 tablespoons cornstarch
- 3 tablespoons stevia
- 2 tablespoons water
- ½ teaspoon cinnamon powder
- 1 teaspoon vanilla extract
- A pinch of nutmeg, ground

Directions:

1. In your slow cooker, mix the carrots with the butter, peach, stevia, cinnamon, vanilla, nutmeg and cornstarch mixed with water, toss, cover and cook on Low for 6 hours.
2. Toss the carrots one more time, divide between plates and serve as a side dish.

Nutrition Info:

Calories139, Fat 10.7g, Cholesterol 0mg, Sodium 199mg, Carbohydrate 35.4g, Fiber 4.2g, Sugars 6.9g, Protein 3.8g, Potassium 25mg

Oregano And Lemon Vegetables

Servings: 6

Cooking Time: 4 Hours

Ingredients:

- 5 carrots, sliced
- 5 ounces baby spinach
- 1 avocado, pitted, peeled and chopped
- 1 yellow onion, chopped
- A pinch of black pepper
- 2 garlic cloves, minced
- ½ teaspoon oregano, dried
- 2 and ½ cups low-sodium veggie stock
- 2 teaspoons lemon peel, grated
- 3 tablespoons lemon juice

Directions:

1. In your slow cooker, mix onion, carrots, garlic, pepper, oregano and stock, stir, cover and cook on High for 4 hours.
2. Add spinach, lemon juice and lemon peel, stir, leave aside for 5 minutes, divide between plates, sprinkle avocado on top and serve as a side dish.

Nutrition Info:

Calories 112, Fat 6.7g, Cholesterol 0mg, Sodium 116mg, Carbohydrate 12g, Fiber 4.7g, Sugars 4.2g, Protein 2.1g, Potassium 501mg

Apples And Kraut

Servings: 8 Servings

Ingredients:

- 2 pounds (900 g) sauerkraut
- 2 cups (490 g) applesauce
- 1 cup (160 g) chopped onion
- 1 cup (225 g) brown sugar
- 2 tablespoons (13.4 g) caraway seeds

Directions:

1. Combine ingredients in slow cooker and simmer for 3 or more hours.

Nutrition Info:

Per serving: 174 g water; 187 calories (2% from fat, 3% from protein, 94% from carb); 2 g protein; 1 g total fat; 0 g saturated fat; 0 g monounsaturated fat; 0 g polyunsaturated fat; 47 g carb; 5 g fiber; 40 g sugar; 49 mg phosphorus; 76 mg calcium; 3 mg iron; 763 mg sodium; 379 mg potassium; 34 IU vitamin A; 0 mg ATE vitamin E; 20 mg vitamin C; 0 mg cholesterol

Macaroni And Two Cheeses

Servings: 8 Servings

Ingredients:

- 8 ounces (225 g) elbow macaroni, cooked al dente
- 13 ounces (365 ml) fat-free evaporated milk
- 1 cup (235 ml) skim milk
- ¼ cup (60 ml) egg substitute
- 4 cups (450 g) shredded Cheddar cheese, divided
- ½ teaspoon white pepper
- ¼ cup (25 g) grated Parmesan cheese

Directions:

1. Spray inside of cooker with nonstick cooking spray. Then, in cooker, combine cooked macaroni, evaporated milk, milk, egg substitute, 3 cups (345 g) Cheddar cheese, salt, and pepper. Top with remaining Cheddar and Parmesan cheeses. Cover and cook on low 3 hours.

Nutrition Info:

Per serving: 98 g water; 440 calories (49% from fat, 25% from protein, 27% from carb); 27 g protein; 24 g total fat; 15 g saturated

fat; 7 g monounsaturated fat; 1 g polyunsaturated fat; 29 g carb; 1 g fiber; 6 g sugar; 548 mg phosphorus; 699 mg calcium; 2 mg iron; 544 mg sodium; 367 mg potassium; 947 IU vitamin A; 247 mg ATE vitamin E; 1 mg vitamin C; 75 mg cholesterol

Vegetables For Pasta

Servings: 6 Servings

Ingredients:

- 2 cups (226 g) sliced zucchini
- 16 cherry tomatoes, cut in half
- ½ cup (75 g) sliced green bell pepper
- ½ cup (75 g) sliced red bell pepper
- ¾ cup (120 g) sliced onion
- 4 ounces (115 g) sliced mushrooms
- 1 teaspoons minced garlic
- 1 tablespoon (15 ml) olive oil
- 1 tablespoon (6 g) Italian seasoning
- 8 ounces (225 g) no-salt-added tomato sauce

Directions:

1. Combine all ingredients in slow cooker. Cook on low 6 hours or until vegetables are tender.

Nutrition Info:

Per serving: 132 g water; 70 calories (32% from fat, 13% from protein, 55% from carb); 2 g protein; 3 g total fat; 0 g saturated fat; 2 g monounsaturated fat; 0 g polyunsaturated fat; 11 g carb;

3 g fiber; 4 g sugar; 57 mg phosphorus; 30 mg calcium; 1 mg iron; 11 mg sodium; 497 mg potassium; 966 IU vitamin A; 0 mg ATE vitamin E; 49 mg vitamin C; 0 mg cholesterol

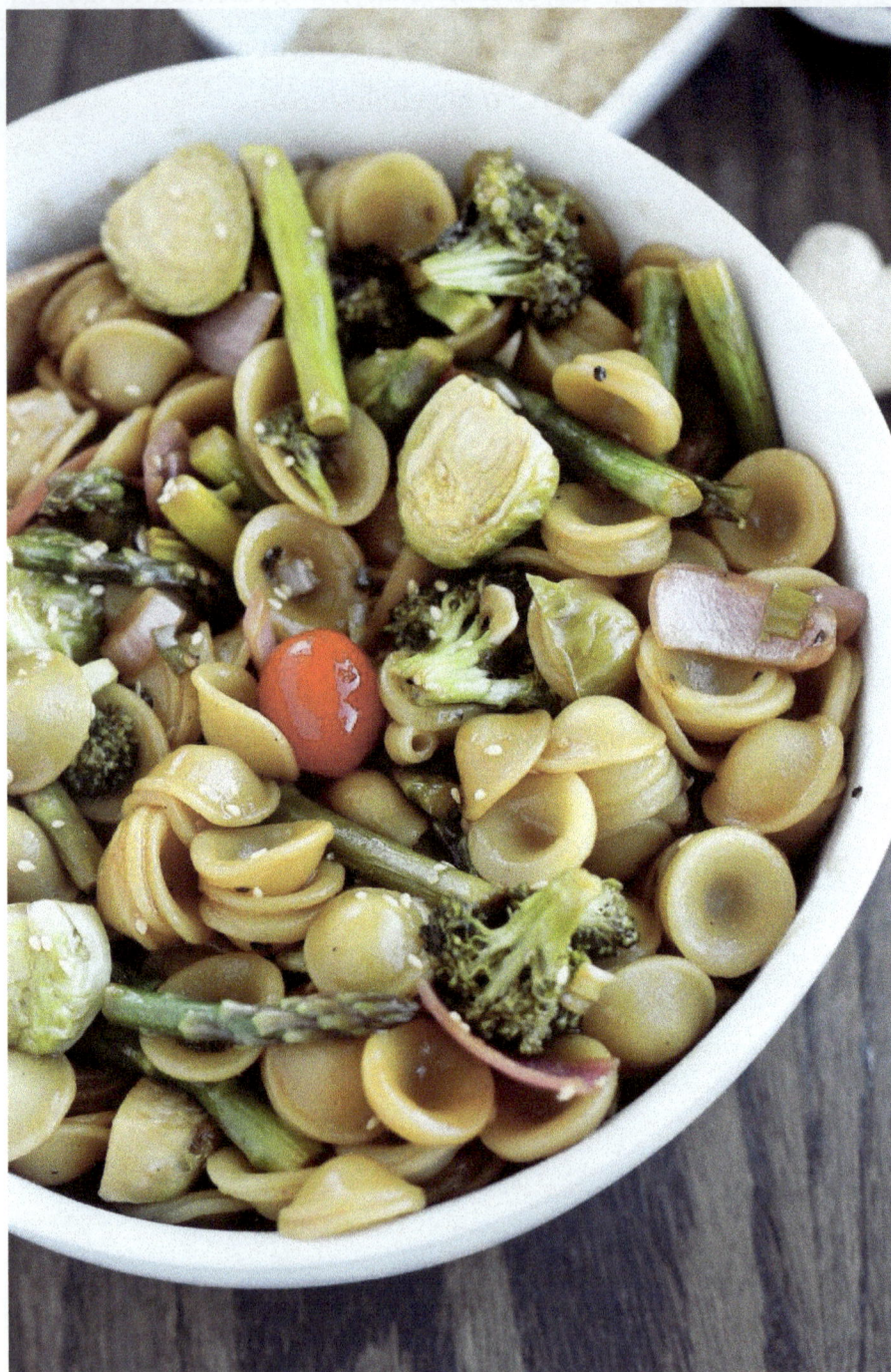

Minced Garlic Cauliflower

Servings: 6

Cooking Time: 3 Hours

Ingredients:

- ½ pound Portobello mushrooms, sliced
- 1 cup cauliflower, riced
- 6 green onions, chopped
- 2 cups water
- 2 garlic cloves, minced
- 3 tablespoons olive oil
- A pinch of black pepper

Directions:

1. In your slow cooker, mix cauliflower with green onions, oil, garlic, mushrooms, water and pepper, stir well, cover, cook on Low for 3 hours, divide between plates and serve as a side dish.

Nutrition Info:

Calories 81, Fat 7.1g, Cholesterol 0mg, Sodium 10mg, Carbohydrate 3.4g, Fiber 0.8g, Sugars 0.8g, Protein 1.7g, Potassium 237mg

Artichoke And Spinach Dip

Servings: About 2

Cooking Time: 2 Hrs 10 Mins

Ingredients:

- 1/8 tsp. Basil (dried)
- 14 oz. chopped Artichoke Hearts
- 1 ½ cups Spinach
- ½ minced clove Garlic
- ¼ cup Sour Cream (low fat)
- ¼ cup shredded Cheese (Parmesan)
- ¼ cup Mozzarella Cheese (shredded)
- 1/8 tsp. Parsley (dried)
- ½ cup Yogurt (Greek)
- Pinch of Black Pepper
- Pinch of Kosher Salt

Directions:

1. Boil spinach in water for 1 min.
2. Drain the water. Set the spinach aside to cool and then chop.
3. Puree all the ingredients including spinach in a blender.

4. Transfer the mixture to the slow cooker.

5. Add cheeses and cook for 1 hour on "low".

6. Serve with sliced vegetables.

Nutrition Info:

(Estimated Amount Per Serving): 263 Calories; 14 g Total Fats; 537 mg Sodium; 42 mg Cholesterol; 18 g Carbohydrates; 6 g Dietary Fiber; 20 g Protein

Fragrant Thyme Mushrooms

Servings: 4

Cooking Time: 4 Hours

Ingredients:

- 4 garlic cloves, minced
- 24 ounces white mushrooms, halved
- 1 teaspoon basil, dried
- 1 teaspoon oregano, dried
- 2 tablespoons olive oil
- 2 tablespoons parsley, chopped
- ¼ teaspoon thyme dried
- 1 cup low-sodium veggie stock
- A pinch of black pepper

Directions:

1. Grease the slow cooker with the oil, add mushrooms, garlic, bay leaves, thyme, basil, oregano, black pepper, parsley and stock, cover, cook on Low for 4 hours, divide between plates and serve as a side dish.

Nutrition Info:

Calories 108, Fat 7.6g, Cholesterol 0mg, Sodium 46mg, Carbohydrate 7.5g, Fiber 2g, Sugars 3.2g, Protein 5.7g, Potassium 571mg

Sweet Butternut

Servings: 8

Cooking Time: 4 Hours

Ingredients:

- 1 cup carrots, chopped
- 1 tablespoon olive oil
- 1 yellow onion, chopped
- ½ teaspoon stevia
- 1 garlic clove, minced
- ½ teaspoon curry powder
- 1 butternut squash, cubed
- 2 and ½ cups low-sodium veggie stock
- ½ cup basmati rice
- ¾ cup coconut milk
- ½ teaspoon cinnamon powder
- ¼ teaspoon ginger, grated

Directions:

1. Heat up a pan with the oil over medium- highheat, add the oil, onion, garlic, stevia, carrots, curry powder, cinnamon and ginger, stir, cook for 5 minutes and transfer to your slow cooker.

2. Add squash, stock and coconut milk, stir, cover and cook on Low for 4 hours.

3. Divide the butternut mix between plates and serve as a side dish.

Nutrition Info:

Calories 134, Fat 7.2g, Cholesterol 0mg, Sodium 59mg, Carbohydrate 16.5g, Fiber 1.7g, Sugars 2.7g, Protein 1.8g, Potassium 202mg

Black Pepper Baby Potatoes

Servings: 12

Cooking Time: 3 Hours

Ingredients:

- 3 pounds baby potatoes, halved
- 7 garlic cloves, minced
- 2 tablespoons olive oil
- 1 tablespoon rosemary, chopped
- A pinch of black pepper

Directions:

1. In your slow cooker, mix oil with potatoes, garlic, rosemary and pepper, toss, cover, cook on High for 3 hours, divide between plates and serve.

Nutrition Info:

Calories 89, Fat 2.5g, Cholesterol 0mg, Sodium 12mg, Carbohydrate 14.9g, Fiber 3g, Sugars 0g, Protein 3g, Potassium 478mg

Caramelized Onions

Servings: 8 Servings

Ingredients:

- 6 large sweet onions, such as Vidalia
- ¼ cup (55 g) unsalted butter
- 1¼ cups (285 ml) low-sodium chicken broth

Directions:

1. Peel onions. Remove stems and root ends. Place in slow cooker. Pour butter and broth over onions. Cook on low 12 hours.

Nutrition Info:

Per serving: 143 g water; 100 calories (51% from fat, 6% from protein, 43% from carb); 2 g protein; 6 g total fat; 4 g saturated fat; 2 g monounsaturated fat; 0 g polyunsaturated fat; 11 g carb; 2 g fiber; 5 g sugar; 40 mg phosphorus; 31 mg calcium; 0 mg iron; 26 mg sodium; 188 mg potassium; 180 IU vitamin A; 48 mg ATE vitamin E; 9 mg vitamin C; 15 mg cholesterol

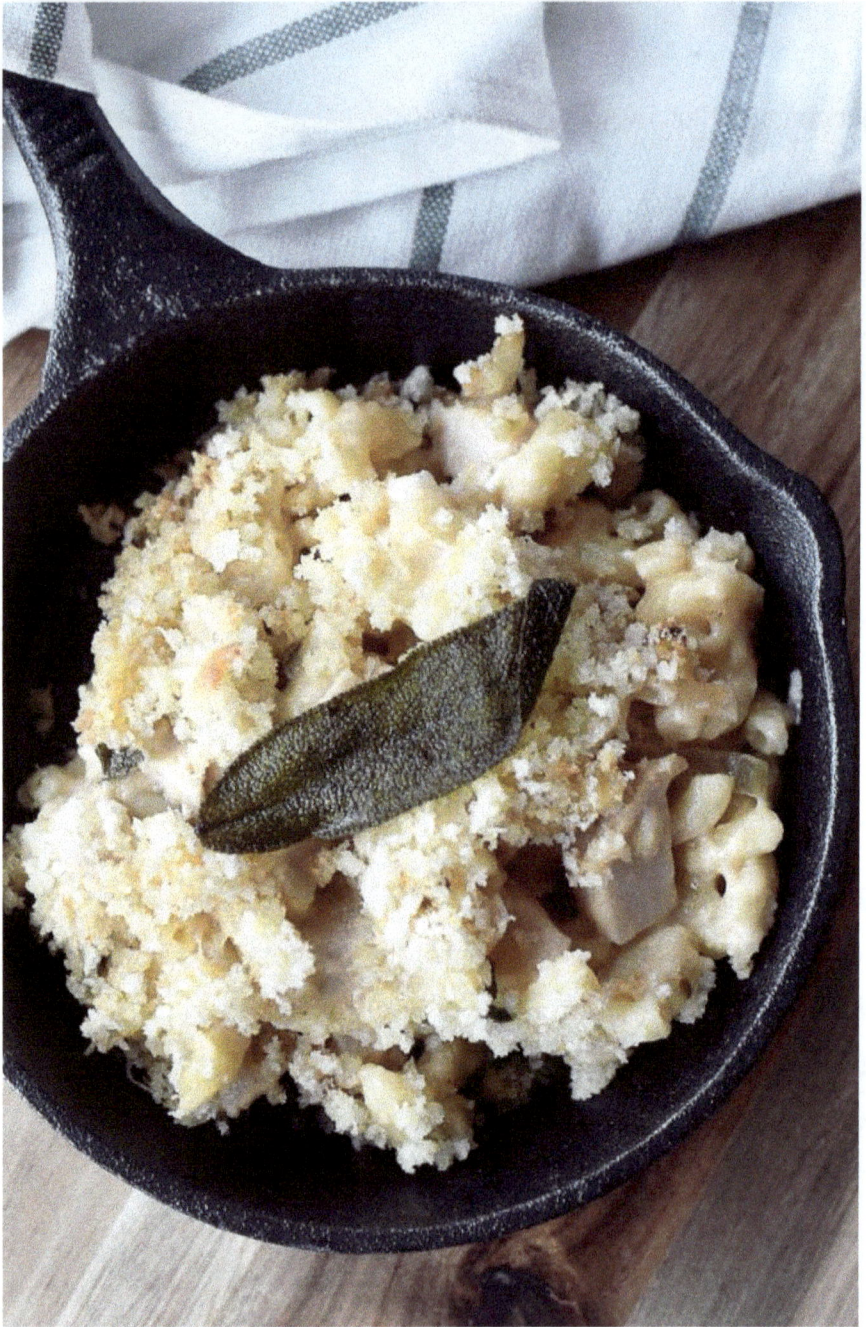

Lemon And Cilantro Rice

Servings: About 4

Cooking Time: 6 Hrs

Ingredients:

- 3 cups Vegetable Broth (low sodium)
- 1 ½ cups Brown Rice (uncooked)
- Juice of2 lemons
- 2 tbsp. chopped Cilantro

Directions:

1. In a slow cooker, place broth and rice.
2. Cook on "low" for 5 hrs.
3. Check the rice for doneness with a fork.
4. Add the lemon juice and cilantro before serving.

Nutrition Info:

(Estimated Amount Per Serving): 56 Calories; 0.3 g Total Fats; 174 mg Sodium; 12 g Carbohydrates; 1 g Dietary Fiber; 1 g Protein

Sour Cream Green Beans

Servings: 8

Cooking Time: 4 Hours

Ingredients:

- 15 ounces green beans
- 14 ounces corn
- 4 ounces mushrooms, sliced
- 11 ounces cream of mushroom soup, low-fat and sodium-free
- ½ cup low-fat sour cream
- ½ cup almonds, chopped
- ½ cup low-fat cheddar cheese, shredded

Directions:

1. In your slow cooker, mix the green beans with the corn, mushrooms soup, mushrooms, almonds, cheese and sour cream, toss, cover and cook on Low for 4 hours.
2. Stir one more time, divide between plates and serve as a side dish.

Nutrition Info:

Calories360, Fat 12.7g, Cholesterol 14mg, Sodium 220mg, Carbohydrate 58.3g, Fiber 10g, Sugars 10.3g, Protein 14g, Potassium 967mg

Vegetable Accompaniment

Servings: 8 Servings

Ingredients:

- 4 potatoes, diced and peeled
- 1¼ cups (205 g) frozen corn
- 2 cups (360 g) seeded and diced tomatoes
- 1 cup (130 g) sliced carrots
- ½ cup (80 g) chopped onion
- ¼ teaspoon dill weed
- ¼ teaspoon black pepper
- ¼ teaspoon basil
- ¼ teaspoon rosemary

Directions:

1. Combine all ingredients in slow cooker. Cover and cook on low 5 to 6 hours or until vegetables are tender.

Nutrition Info:

Per serving: 227 g water; 168 calories (3% from fat, 11% from protein, 87% from carb); 5 g protein; 1 g total fat; 0 g saturated fat; 0 g monounsaturated fat; 0 g polyunsaturated fat; 39 g carb; 5 g fiber; 4 g sugar; 145 mg phosphorus; 30 mg calcium; 2 mg iron; 27 mg sodium; 1028 mg potassium; 2940 IU vitamin A; 0 mg ATE vitamin E; 28 mg vitamin C; 0 mg cholesterol

Curry Eggplant

Servings: 4

Cooking Time: 3 Hours

Ingredients:

- 2 cups cherry tomatoes, halved
- 1 eggplant, sliced
- ½ teaspoon cumin, ground
- 1 teaspoon mustard seed
- ½ teaspoon coriander, ground
- ½ teaspoon curry powder
- A pinch of nutmeg, ground
- ½ yellow onion, chopped
- 1 tablespoon cilantro, chopped
- 1 teaspoon red wine vinegar
- 1 tablespoon olive oil
- 1 garlic clove, minced
- Black pepper to the taste

Directions:

1. Grease the slow cooker with the oil and add eggplant slices inside.

2. Add cumin, mustard seeds, coriander, curry powder, nutmeg, tomatoes, onion, garlic, vinegar, black pepper and cilantro, cover and cook on High for 3 hours.

3. Divide between plates and serve as a side dish.

Nutrition Info:

Calories 94, Fat 4.6g, Cholesterol 0mg, Sodium 64mg, Carbohydrate 13.2g, Fiber 5.7g, Sugars 7g, Protein 2.5g, Potassium 514mg

Coconut Mashed Potatoes

Servings: 6

Cooking Time: 4 Hours

Ingredients:

- 3 pounds gold potatoes, peeled and cubed
- 6 garlic cloves, peeled
- 28 ounces low-sodium veggie stock
- 1 bay leaf
- 1 cup coconut milk
- 3 tablespoons olive oil
- Black pepper to the taste

Directions:

1. In your slow cooker, mix potatoes with stock, bay leaf, garlic, salt and pepper, cover and cook on High for 4 hours.
2. Drain potatoes and garlic, mash them, add oil and milk, whisk well, divide between plates and serve as a side dish.

Nutrition Info:

Calories 321, Fat 16.8g, Cholesterol 0mg, Sodium 121mg, Carbohydrate 41.2g, Fiber 7g, Sugars 5.2g, Protein 4.2g, Potassium 1055mg

Bean Soup

Servings: 4

Cooking Time: 5 Hrs

Ingredients:

- ½ cup Pinto Beans (dried)
- ½ Bay Leaf
- 1 clove Garlic
- ½ Onion (white)
- 2 cups Water
- 2 tbsp. Cilantro (chopped)
- 1 cubed Avocado
- 1/8 cup White Onion (chopped)
- ¼ cup Roma Tomatoes (chopped)
- 2 tbsp. Pepper Sauce (chipotle)
- ¼ tsp. Kosher Salt
- 2 tbsp. chopped Cilantro
- 2 tbsp. Low Fat Monterrey Jack Cheese, shredded

Directions:

1. Place water, salt, onion, pepper, garlic, bay leaf and beans in the slow cooker.
2. Cook on high for 5-6 hours.

3. Discard the Bay leaf.

4. Serve in heated bowls.

Nutrition Info:

(Estimated Amount Per Serving): 258 Calories; 19 g Total Fats; 2 mg Cholesterol; 620 mg Sodium; 25 mg Carbohydrates; 11 g Dietary Fiber; 8 g Protein

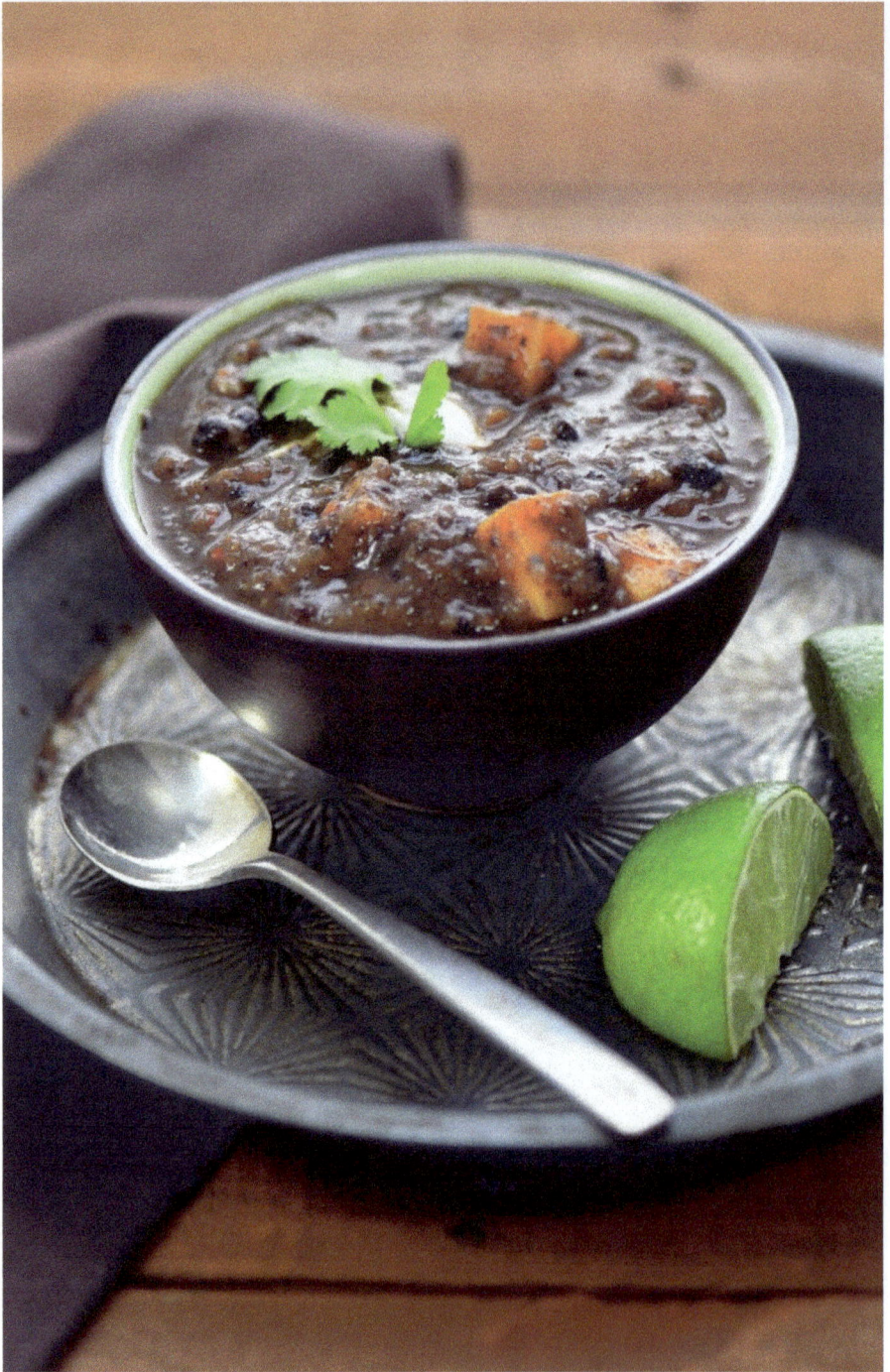

White Chili

Servings: 8 Servings

Ingredients:

- 6 cups (1.1 kg) great northern beans, cooked or canned without salt, drained
- 8 ounces (225 g) shredded cooked chicken breasts
- 1 cup (160 g) chopped onion
- 1½ cups (225 g) chopped green bell pepper
- 4 ounces (115 g) diced green chilies
- ¾ teaspoon minced garlic
- 2 teaspoons cumin
- ½ teaspoon oregano
- 3½ cups (820 ml) low-sodium chicken broth

Directions:

1. Combine all ingredients in slow cooker. Cover and cook on low 8 to 10 hours or on high 4 to 5 hours.

Nutrition Info:

Per serving: 317 g water; 290 calories (6% from fat, 32% from protein, 62% from carb); 24 g protein; 2 g total fat; 1 g saturated fat; 0 g monounsaturated fat; 1 g polyunsaturated fat; 46 g carb;

11 g fiber; 2 g sugar; 342 mg phosphorus; 131 mg calcium; 4 mg iron; 146 mg sodium; 879 mg potassium; 138 IU vitamin A; 2 mg ATE vitamin E; 31 mg vitamin C; 22 mg cholesterol

Chicken Corn Soup

Servings: 6 Servings

Ingredients:

- 1 pound (455 g) boneless skinless chicken breast, cubed
- 1 cup (160 g) chopped onion
- ½ teaspoon minced garlic
- ¾ cup (98 g) sliced carrots
- ½ cup (50 g) chopped celery
- 2 medium potatoes, cubed
- 12 ounces (340 g) cream-style corn
- 12 ounces (340 g) frozen corn
- 2 cups (475 ml) low-sodium chicken broth
- ¼ teaspoon pepper

Directions:

1. Combine all ingredients in slow cooker. Cover and cook on low 8 to 9 hours or until chicken is tender.

Nutrition Info:

Per serving: 369 g water; 278 calories (6% from fat, 32% from protein, 62% from carb); 23 g protein; 2 g total fat; 0 g saturated

fat; 0 g monounsaturated fat; 1 g polyunsaturated fat; 45 g carb; 5 g fiber; 7 g sugar; 309 mg phosphorus; 43 mg calcium; 2 mg iron; 127 mg sodium; 1049 mg potassium; 2800 IU vitamin A; 5 mg ATE vitamin E; 19 mg vitamin C; 44 mg cholesterol

Squash And Bean Soup

Servings: 6 Servings

Ingredients:

- 1 cup (160 g) chopped onion
- 1 tablespoon (15 ml) olive oil
- ½ teaspoon ground cumin
- ¼ teaspoon cinnamon
- ½ teaspoon minced garlic
- 3 cups (420 g) butternut squash, peeled and cut into 1-inch (2.5 cm) cubes
- 1½ cups (355 ml) low-sodium vegetable broth
- 2 cups (450 g) great northern beans, cooked or canned without salt
- 1 can (14 ounces, or 400 g) no-salt-added diced tomatoes, undrained
- 1 tablespoon chopped fresh cilantro

Directions:

1. Combine all ingredients in slow cooker. Cover and cook on high 1 hour. Reduce heat to low and cook 2 to 3 hours.

Nutrition Info:

Per serving: 267 g water; 184 calories (15% from fat, 19% from protein, 66% from carb); 9 g protein; 3 g total fat; 1 g saturated fat; 2 g monounsaturated fat; 1 g polyunsaturated fat; 32 g carb; 7 g fiber; 4 g sugar; 182 mg phosphorus; 128 mg calcium; 3 mg iron; 52 mg sodium; 776 mg potassium; 7553 IU vitamin A; 1 mg ATE vitamin E; 24 mg vitamin C; 0 mg cholesterol

Chinese Pork Soup

Servings: 6 Servings

Ingredients:

- 1 pound (455 g) boneless pork loin roast, cut in ½–inch (1.3 cm) cubes
- 1 cup (130 g) julienned carrots
- ½ cup (50 g) chopped scallions
- ½ teaspoon finely chopped garlic
- ¼ cup (60 ml) low-sodium soy sauce
- ½ teaspoon finely chopped fresh ginger
- ¼ teaspoon black pepper
- 2 cups (475 ml) low-sodium beef broth
- 4 ounces (115 g) mushrooms, sliced
- 1 cup (50 g) bean sprouts

Directions:

1. Cook pork in large nonstick skillet over medium heat for 8 to 10 minutes. Stir occasionally. Mix pork and remaining ingredients except mushrooms and bean sprouts in slow cooker. Cover and cook on low 7 to 9 hours or on high 3 to 4 hours. Stir in mushrooms and bean sprouts. Cover and cook on low 1 hour.

Nutrition Info:

Per serving: 204 g water; 145 calories (33% from fat, 54% from protein, 13% from carb); 19 g protein; 5 g total fat; 2 g saturated fat; 2 g monounsaturated fat; 1 g polyunsaturated fat; 5 g carb; 1 g fiber; 2 g sugar; 213 mg phosphorus; 28 mg calcium; 1 mg iron; 160 mg sodium; 540 mg potassium; 3677 IU vitamin A; 2 mg ATE vitamin E; 4 mg vitamin C; 42 mg cholesterol

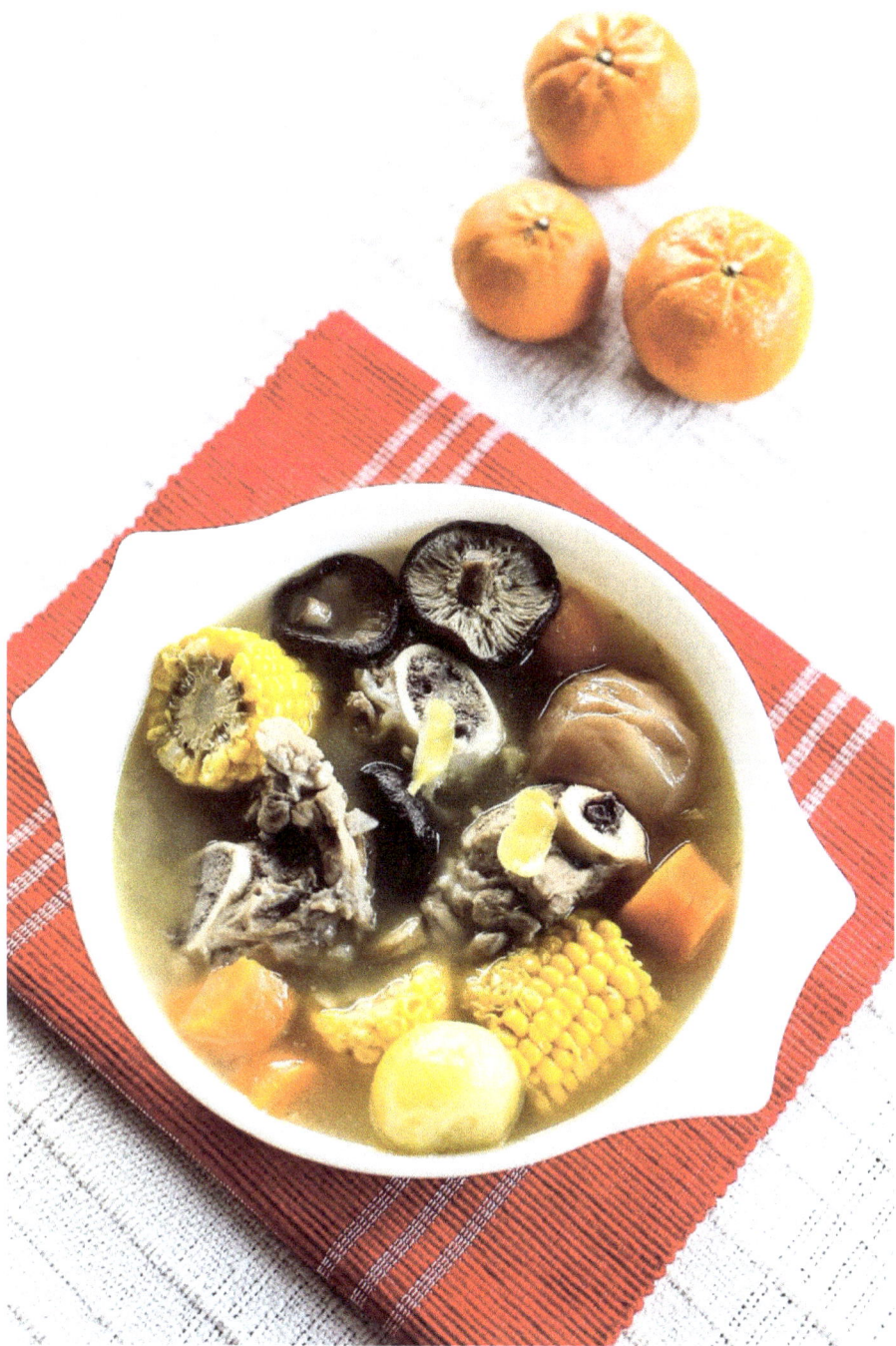

Vegetarian Minestrone

Servings: 6 Servings

Ingredients:

- 6 cups (1.4 L) low-sodium vegetable broth
- ¾ cup (98 g) chopped carrots
- 1½ cup (240 g) chopped onions
- 1/3 cup (33 g) chopped celery
- ½ teaspoon minced garlic
- ½ cup (60 g) cubed zucchini
- 1 cup (67 g) chopped kale
- ½ cup (100 g) pearl barley
- 2 cups (480 g) canned no-salt-added chickpeas, drained
- 1 tablespoon (1.3 g) parsley
- ½ teaspoon thyme
- 1 teaspoon oregano
- 1 can (28 ounces, or 785 g) no-salt-added crushed tomatoes
- ¼ teaspoon pepper

Directions:

1. Combine all ingredients in slow cooker. Cover and cook on low 6 to 8 hours or until vegetables are tender.

Nutrition Info:

Per serving: 469 g water; 238 calories (13% from fat, 22% from protein, 64% from carb); 14 g protein; 4 g total fat; 1 g saturated fat; 1 g monounsaturated fat; 1 g polyunsaturated fat; 40 g carb; 10 g fiber; 9 g sugar; 261 mg phosphorus; 185 mg calcium; 5 mg iron; 186 mg sodium; 896 mg potassium; 4708 IU vitamin A; 2 mg ATE vitamin E; 33 mg vitamin C; 0 mg cholesterol

Broccoli Soup

Servings: About 2

Cooking Time: 3 Hrs

Ingredients:

- 4 cups chopped Broccoli
- ½ cup chopped Onion (white)
- 1 ½ cup Chicken Broth (low sodium)
- 1/8 tsp. Black Pepper (cracked)
- 1 tbsp. Olive Oil
- 1 Garlic Clove
- 1/16 tsp. Pepper Flakes (chili)
- ¼ cup Milk (low fat)

Directions:

1. In the slow cooker, cover the broccoli with water and cook for an hour on "high."
2. Set aside after draining.
3. Sauté onion and garlic in oil and transfer them to slow cooker when done.
4. Add the broth.
5. Cook on "low" for 2 hrs.

6. Transfer the mixture to a blender and make a smooth puree. Add black pepper, milk and pepper flakes to the puree.
7. Boil briefly.
8. Serve the soup in heated bowls.

Nutrition Info:

(Estimated Amount Per Serving): 291 Calories; 14 g Total Fats; 24 mg Cholesterol; 227 mg Sodium; 28 mg Carbohydrates; 6 g Dietary Fiber; 17 g Protein

Tomato Soup

Servings: 6 Servings

Ingredients:

- 5 cups (1.2 L) diced tomatoes
- 1 tablespoon (16 g) no-salt-added tomato paste
- 4 cups (950 ml) low-sodium vegetable broth
- ½ cup (80 g) minced onion
- 1 tablespoon (10 g) minced garlic
- 1 teaspoon basil
- ¼ teaspoon black pepper

Directions:

1. Combine all ingredients in a slow cooker. Cook on low for 6 to 8 hours. Stir once while cooking.

Nutrition Info:

Per serving: 287 g water; 62 calories (19% from fat, 28% from protein, 53% from carb); 5 g protein; 1 g total fat; 0 g saturated fat; 0 g monounsaturated fat; 0 g polyunsaturated fat; 9 g carb; 2 g fiber; 1 g sugar; 88 mg phosphorus; 64 mg calcium; 1 mg iron; 108 mg sodium; 473 mg potassium; 833 IU vitamin A; 2 mg ATE vitamin E; 34 mg vitamin C; 0 mg cholesterol

Cauliflower Soup

Servings: 6 Servings

Ingredients:

- 4 cups (400 g) diced cauliflower
- 2 cups (475 ml) water
- 8 ounces (225 g) fat-free cream cheese
- ½ cup (60 g) shredded Cheddar
- ½ cup (30 g) potato flakes

Directions:

1. Combine cauliflower and water in a saucepan. Heat to boiling. Places cheeses in slow cooker. Stir in cauliflower and water. Mix well. Stir in potato flakes and cook on low for 2 to 3 hours.

Nutrition Info:

Per serving: 184 g water; 168 calories (56% from fat, 20% from protein, 24% from carb); 9 g protein; 11 g total fat; 7 g saturated fat; 3 g monounsaturated fat; 1 g polyunsaturated fat; 10 g carb; 2 g fiber; 2 g sugar; 146 mg phosphorus; 139 mg calcium; 1 mg iron; 200 mg sodium; 247 mg potassium; 377 IU vitamin A; 97 mg ATE vitamin E; 41 mg vitamin C; 33 mg cholesterol

Brunswick Stew

Servings: 10 Servings

Ingredients:

- 3 potatoes, peeled and cut in ½-inch (1.3 cm) pieces
- 10 ounces (280 g) frozen lima beans
- 10 ounces (280 g) frozen okra
- 10 ounces (280 g) frozen corn
- 3 cups (420 g) diced cooked chicken breast
- 1 tablespoon (13 g) sugar
- ½ teaspoon rosemary
- ¼ teaspoon black pepper
- ¼ teaspoon cloves
- 1 bay leaf
- 4 cups (950 ml) low-sodium chicken broth
- 1 can (14 ounces, or 400 g) no-salt-added whole peeled tomatoes, cut up

Directions:

1. Place potatoes and frozen vegetables in slow cooker. Add chicken, sugar, rosemary, pepper, cloves, and bay leaf. Pour chicken broth and undrained tomatoes over

mixture. Cover and cook on low for 8 to 10 hours. Remove bay leaf and stir well before serving.

Nutrition Info:

Per serving: 297 g water; 203 calories (9% from fat, 36% from protein, 56% from carb); 18 g protein; 2 g total fat; 1 g saturated fat; 1 g monounsaturated fat; 0 g polyunsaturated fat; 29 g carb; 5 g fiber; 4 g sugar; 233 mg phosphorus; 65 mg calcium; 3 mg iron; 110 mg sodium; 923 mg potassium; 218 IU vitamin A; 3 mg ATE vitamin E; 21 mg vitamin C; 36 mg cholesterol

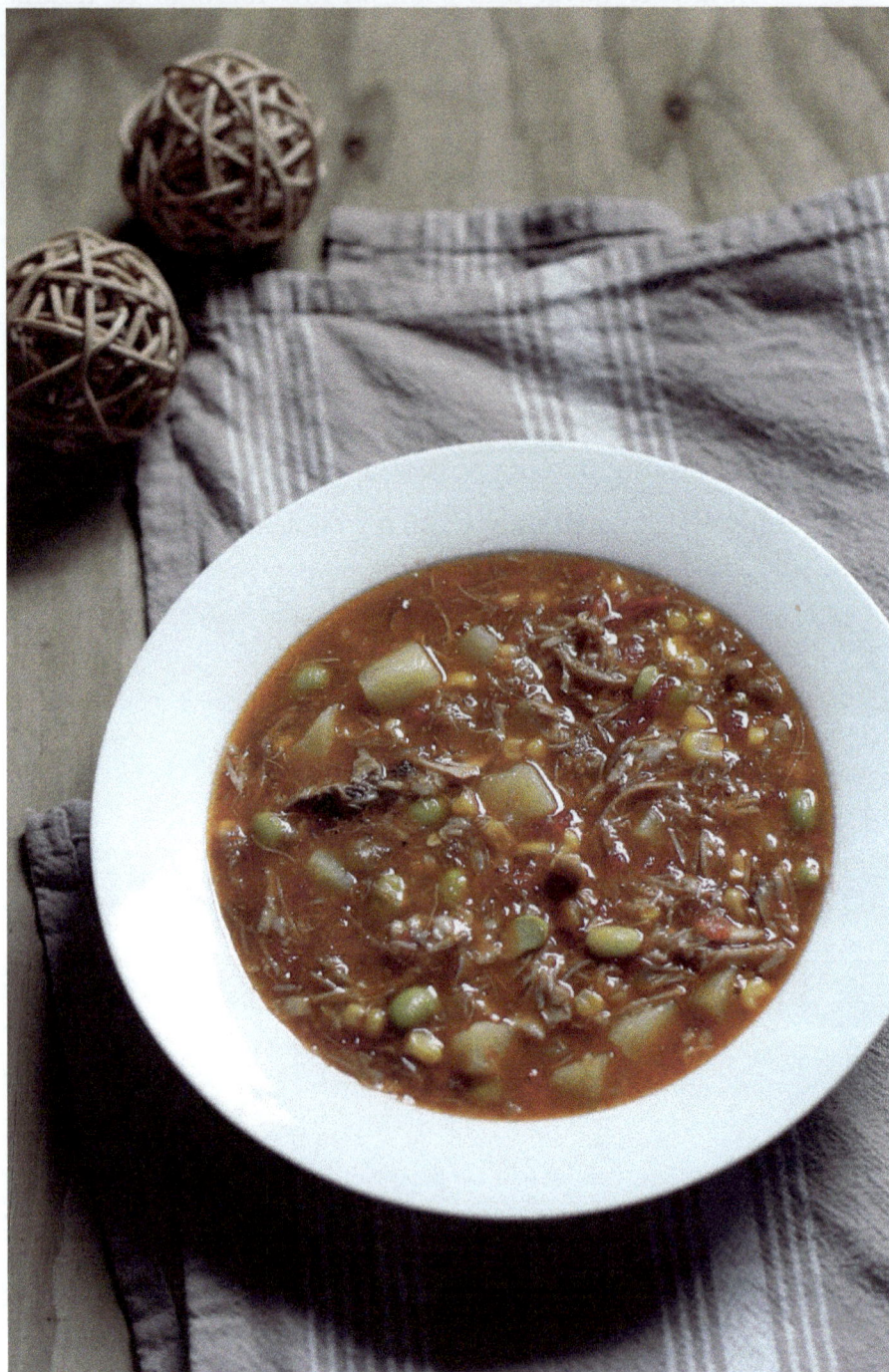

Black Bean Chili

Servings: 8 Serving s

Ingredients:

- 1 pound (455 g) pork loin, cut in 1-inch (2.5 cm) cubes
- 2 cups (520 g) low-sodium salsa
- 4 cups (688 g) black beans, cooked or canned without salt
- ½ cup (120 ml) low-sodium chicken broth
- 1 cup (150 g) chopped red bell peppers
- 1 cup (160 g) chopped onion
- 1 teaspoon cumin
- 2 tablespoons (15 g) chili powder
- 1 teaspoon oregano

Directions:

1. Brown pork in skillet over medium-high heat. Drain. Combine pork and remaining ingredients in slow cooker. Cover and cook on low 8 to 10 hours.

Nutrition Info:

Per serving: 196 g water; 221 calories (14% from fat, 37% from protein, 49% from carb); 21 g protein; 3 g total fat; 1 g saturated

fat; 1 g monounsaturated fat; 1 g polyunsaturated fat; 28 g carb; 10 g fiber; 3 g sugar; 280 mg phosphorus; 61 mg calcium; 3 mg iron; 183 mg sodium; 788 mg potassium; 1316 IU vitamin A; 1 mg ATE vitamin E; 28 mg vitamin C; 36 mg cholesterol

Pasta And Bean Soup

Servings: 6 Servings

Ingredients:

- 1 cup (180 g) chopped tomatoes
- ½ cup (75 g) uncooked macaroni
- ½ cup (80 g) chopped onion
- ¼ cup (40 g) chopped green bell pepper
- 1 teaspoon basil
- 1 teaspoon Worcestershire sauce
- ½ teaspoon chopped garlic
- 1 can (15 ounces, or 420 g) no-salt-added kidney beans, drained
- 1 can (15 ounces, or 420 g) no-salt-added chickpeas, drained
- 2 cups (475 ml) low-sodium vegetable broth

Directions:

1. Combine all ingredients in slow cooker. Cook on low 5 to 6 hours.

Nutrition Info:

Per serving: 224 g water; 216 calories (7% from fat, 24% from protein, 70% from carb); 13 g protein; 2 g total fat; 0 g saturated fat; 0 g monounsaturated fat; 1 g polyunsaturated fat; 38 g carb; 11 g fiber; 1 g sugar; 208 mg phosphorus; 87 mg calcium; 4 mg iron; 273 mg sodium; 562 mg potassium; 212 IU vitamin A; 1 mg ATE vitamin E; 18 mg vitamin C; 0 mg cholesterol

4-WEEK MEAL PLAN

Week 1

Monday
Breakfast: Tofu Frittata
Lunch: Pork Chops In Beer
Dinner: Stewed Tomatoes

Tuesday
Breakfast: Tapioca
Lunch: Creamy Beef Burgundy
Dinner: Oregano Salad

Wednesday
Breakfast: Fruit Oats
Lunch: Smothered Steak
Dinner: Black Beans With Corn Kernels

Thursday
Breakfast: Grapefruit Mix
Lunch: Pork For Sandwiches
Dinner: Stuffed Acorn Squash

Friday
Breakfast: Berry Yogurt
Lunch: Cranberry Pork Roast

Dinner: Greek Eggplant

Saturday
Breakfast: Soft Pudding
Lunch: Pan-asian Pot Roast
Dinner: Thyme Sweet Potatoes

Sunday
Breakfast: Black Beans Salad
Lunch: Short Ribs
Dinner: Barley Vegetable Soup

Week 2

Monday
Breakfast: Carrot Pudding
Lunch: French Dip
Dinner: Butter Corn

Tuesday
Breakfast: Apple Cake
Lunch: Italian Roast With Vegetables
Dinner: Orange Glazed Carrots

Wednesday
Breakfast: Almond Milk Barley Cereals
Lunch: Honey Mustard Ribs
Dinner: Cinnamon Acorn Squash

Thursday
Breakfast: Cashews Cake
Lunch: Pizza Casserole
Dinner: Glazed Root Vegetables

Friday
Breakfast: Artichoke Frittata
Lunch: Hawaiian Pork Roast
Dinner: Stir Fried Steak, Shiitake And Asparagus

Saturday
Breakfast: Mexican Eggs
Lunch: Apple Cranberry Pork Roast
Dinner: Cilantro Brussel Sprouts

Sunday
Breakfast: Stewed Peach
Lunch: Swiss Steak
Dinner: Italian Zucchini

Week 3

Monday
Breakfast: Lamb Cassoule t
Lunch: Glazed Pork Roast
Dinner: Cilantro Parsnip Chunks

Tuesday

Breakfast: Fruited Tapioca

Lunch: Swiss Steak In Wine Sauce

Dinner: Corn Casserole

Wednesday

Breakfast: Baby Spinach Shrimp Salad

Lunch: Italian Pork Chops

Dinner: Pilaf With Bella Mushrooms

Thursday

Breakfast: Coconut And Fruit Cake

Lunch: Italian Pot Roast

Dinner: Italian Style Yellow Squash

Friday

Breakfast: Apple And Squash Bowls

Lunch: Beef With Horseradish Sauce

Dinner: Stevia Peas With Marjoram

Saturday

Breakfast: Slow Cooker Chocolate Cake

Lunch: Oriental Pot Roast

Dinner: Broccoli Rice Casserole

Sunday

Breakfast: Fish Omelet

Lunch: Barbecued Ribs

Dinner: Italians Style Mushroom Mix

Week 4

Monday
Breakfast: Brown Cake
Lunch: Ham And Scalloped Pota toes
Dinner: Broccoli Casserole

Tuesday
Breakfast: Stevia And Walnuts Cut Oats
Lunch: Pork And Pineapple Roast

Wednesday
Breakfast: Walnut And Cinnamon Oatmeal
Lunch: Barbecued Brisket
Dinner: Dinner: Slow Cooker Lasagna

Thursday
Breakfast: Tender Rosemary Sweet Potatoes
Lunch: Barbecued Short Ribs
Dinner: Brussels Sprouts Casserole

Friday
Breakfast: Orange And Maple Syrup Quinoa
Lunch: Beer-braised Short Ribs
Dinner: Pasta And Mushrooms

Saturday
Breakfast: Vanilla And Nutmeg Oatmeal
Lunch: Lamb Stew
Dinner: Onion Cabbage

Sunday

Breakfast: Pecans Cake

Lunch: Barbecued Ham

Dinner: Cheese Broccoli

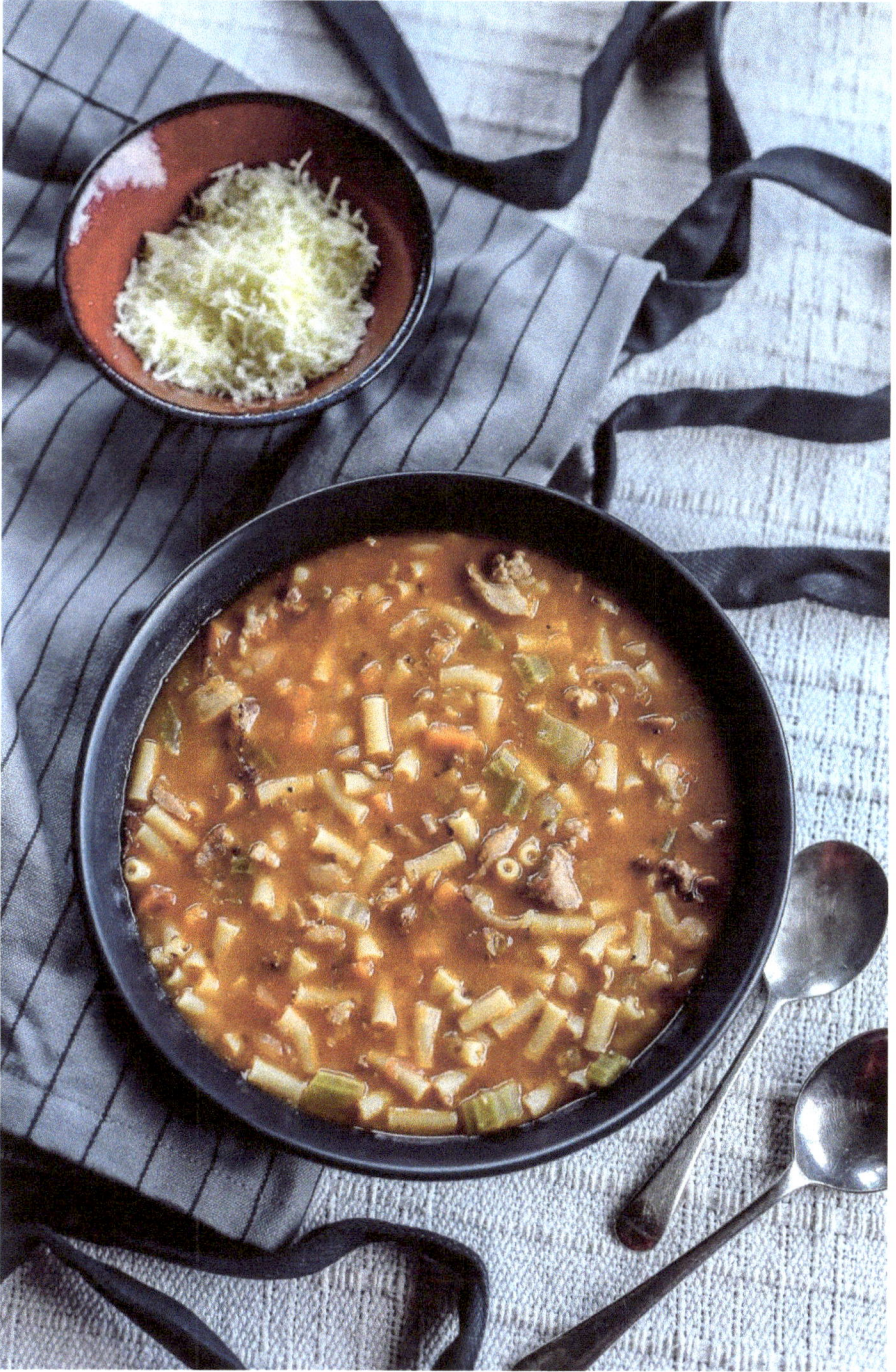

Lightning Source UK Ltd.
Milton Keynes UK
UKHW020815170621
385664UK00001B/163

9 781802 778526